Essential Oils Diffuser:

Top 40 Essential Oil Recipes

Table of content

Introduction

It was another long day at the office, and all you want to do is get home and settle in for the evening. You want to relax, enjoy yourself, and have a good time for a while before you have to get the rest of your day underway.

What is the best way to create the atmosphere you want?

To infuse the air with all kinds of delicious scents that make you feel wonderful. There are a number of different options for you to choose from, whether you want to burn an incense, melt a wax cube, or go with plug in methods.

But, while there are a number of things for you to consider, you aren't going to find a better option than going with essential oils. Essential oils are entirely natural, they don't require that you use flame or other hazardous items, and they are perfect to use in any room of the house.

Essential oils are the perfect choice if you want to use something that is not only delicious and natural, but something that is going to help you in your day, too!

"I like scents, but I don't want to have to supervise the room for hours."

"I love wonderful smells, but I don't like the headache that I get when I am around them for extended periods."

"Those melts and waxes are expensive, and I don't want to have to worry about the cost of the melt every time I want to relax."

These are just a few of the many different reasons you want to avoid other scented items. But, when it comes to essential oils, you are going to not only save money, enjoy a safe scent, and be able to relax knowing you are using something entirely natural, but it is also going to aid in any ailment you feel.

Say goodbye to the stress and headaches the natural way and save money while you do. There are so many benefits that come from the use of essential oils, you are going to love each and every one of them.

So go ahead, indulge a little.

Chapter 1 – Good Mood Blends

In this book you are going to find all kinds of blends. You are going to find those that are fruity, those that embrace the wild side of the world, and those that grasp the musk and all of the natural scents that you simply must love.

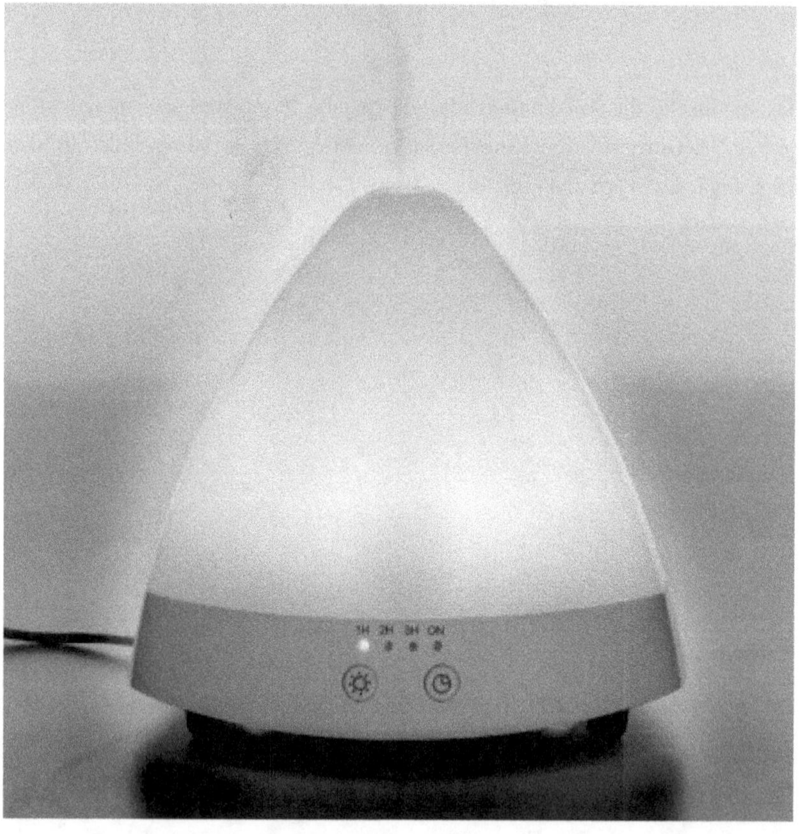

https://www.google.com/search?q=diffuser&espv=2&biw=1366&bih=667&site=webhp&source=lnms&tbm=isch&sa=X&ved=0ahUKEwi2ybOGjvLNAhUHLmMKHbomCEMQ_AUIBygC#imgrc=Rptq34BLaMbFyM%3A

I want you to love each and every blend in this book, and by the time you work your way through all of the recipes, I want you to be in love with your diffuser as though it were one of your best friends in and of itself.

I don't ever want you to feel as though you are doing it wrong, or that you need something different to be happy with your oils. No matter what kind of diffuser you have, what kind of place you live in, or what your favorite scents are, this is the book that is for you.

Use these recipes as they are, use them for inspiration, or combine the two, but no matter what you do, have fun with it and fall in love with the finished product you craft.

The more happiness you feel as you blend, the more happiness is going to come out as you diffuse, and the better you are going to feel in your home. So grab that diffuser, and sit down with some tea, you are going to make happiness in a bottle as easy as one, two, three.

Sunshine Blend

5 drops lavender

5 drops hibiscus

5 drops lemongrass

Combine all the oils together in a glass jar, or directly into your diffuser. Fill your diffuser with water according to the size of your diffuser.

You can follow the recipe here as is, or you can feel free to modify to your own personal preference. Whatever you decide to do, have fun with it and love your blend!

Good Day Blend

5 drops rosewood

3 drops lemon

3 drops lemongrass

Combine all the oils together in a glass jar, or directly into your diffuser. Fill your diffuser with water according to the size of your diffuser.

You can follow the recipe here as is, or you can feel free to modify to your own personal preference. Whatever you decide to do, have fun with it and love your blend!

The Candyshop Blend

5 drops peppermint

3 drops lemon

3 drops rose

1 drop lavender

Combine all the oils together in a glass jar, or directly into your diffuser. Fill your diffuser with water according to the size of your diffuser.

You can follow the recipe here as is, or you can feel free to modify to your own personal preference. Whatever you decide to do, have fun with it and love your blend!

Money for my Honey

6 drops goldenseal

5 drops frankincense

3 drops rosewood

Combine all the oils together in a glass jar, or directly into your diffuser. Fill your diffuser with water according to the size of your diffuser.

You can follow the recipe here as is, or you can feel free to modify to your own personal preference. Whatever you decide to do, have fun with it and love your blend!

Fluffy Clouds

8 drops myrrh

5 drops goldenseal

3 drops orange

Combine all the oils together in a glass jar, or directly into your diffuser. Fill your diffuser with water according to the size of your diffuser.

You can follow the recipe here as is, or you can feel free to modify to your own personal preference. Whatever you decide to do, have fun with it and love your blend!

Peaceful Blend

8 drops agar

5 drops anise

5 drops rose

Combine all the oils together in a glass jar, or directly into your diffuser. Fill your diffuser with water according to the size of your diffuser.

You can follow the recipe here as is, or you can feel free to modify to your own personal preference. Whatever you decide to do, have fun with it and love your blend!

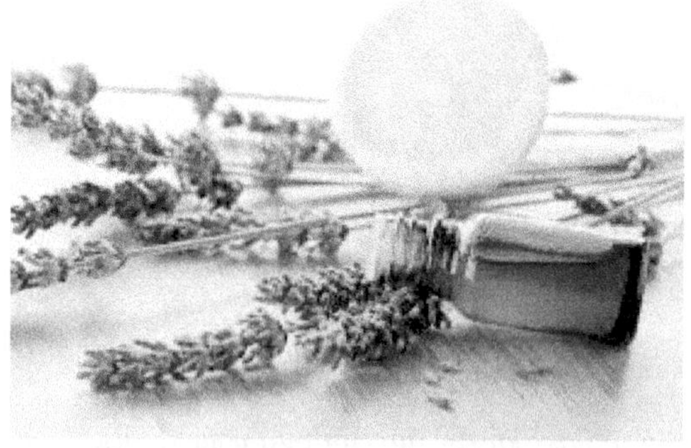

Thankfulness

8 drops bergamot

8 drops lime

5 drops lilac

Combine all the oils together in a glass jar, or directly into your diffuser. Fill your diffuser with water according to the size of your diffuser.

You can follow the recipe here as is, or you can feel free to modify to your own personal preference. Whatever you decide to do, have fun with it and love your blend!

Smiles and Laughter

8 drops anise

8 drops geranium

5 drops black pepper

Combine all the oils together in a glass jar, or directly into your diffuser. Fill your diffuser with water according to the size of your diffuser.

You can follow the recipe here as is, or you can feel free to modify to your own personal preference. Whatever you decide to do, have fun with it and love your blend!

Chapter 2 – All The Spice And Twice As Nice

When you think of happiness and the scents that go along with the feeling, you may start to think of such things as parties, beaches, fairs, the ocean, and things along those lines.

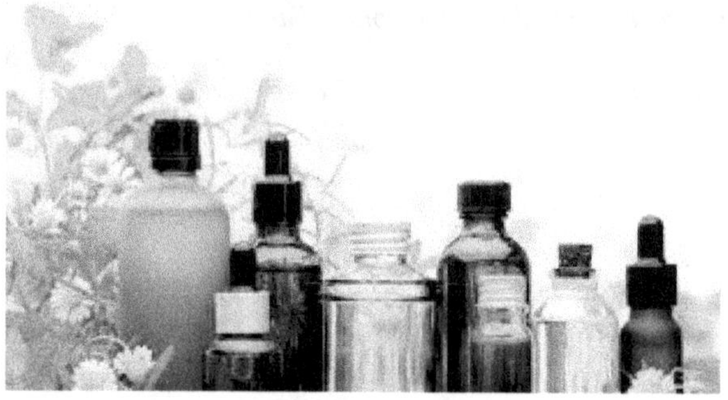

https://www.google.com/search?q=diffuser&espv=2&biw=1366&bih=667&site=webhp&source=lnms&tbm=isch&sa=X&ved=0ahUKEwi2ybOGjvLNAhUHLmMKHbomCEMQ_AUIBygC#imgrc=Rptq34BLaMbFyM%3A

And there is nothing at all wrong with that, those are all incredible places to go and fun things to do, and they are more often than not the things most associate with good feelings, but I want to challenge you to take a step out of the norm.

Don't think that you have to be at the beach to have fun, but embrace the world around you. Think of the dark, musky scents that the earth brings. Go out into your garden, into the fields, and into anywhere you can think of where you can breathe in the rustic smell of trees, dust, and soil.

You are going to find a whole new level of happiness you never thought of before, and you will want to capture that scent for your own home.

With these blends, you are going to get a glimpse of that musk anywhere in your house that you want, and anytime you want, you can escape to that happy place where you embrace nature for all that it is.

And you will never want to walk away.

Arabian Nights

8 drops sandalwood

5 drops myrrh

5 drops patchouli

Combine all the oils together in a glass jar, or directly into your diffuser. Fill your diffuser with water according to the size of your diffuser.

You can follow the recipe here as is, or you can feel free to modify to your own personal preference. Whatever you decide to do, have fun with it and love your blend!

Spice Girl Life Blend

10 drops cinnamon

5 drops ginger

5 drops sandalwood

Combine all the oils together in a glass jar, or directly into your diffuser. Fill your diffuser with water according to the size of your diffuser.

You can follow the recipe here as is, or you can feel free to modify to your own personal preference. Whatever you decide to do, have fun with it and love your blend!

Magic Musky Moonlight

8 drops cardamom

7 drops cedar

7 drops chamomile

Combine all the oils together in a glass jar, or directly into your diffuser. Fill your diffuser with water according to the size of your diffuser.

You can follow the recipe here as is, or you can feel free to modify to your own personal preference. Whatever you decide to do, have fun with it and love your blend!

The Dessert Spice Blend

6 drops clary sage

8 drops sandalwood

5 drops calamus

Combine all the oils together in a glass jar, or directly into your diffuser. Fill your diffuser with water according to the size of your diffuser.

You can follow the recipe here as is, or you can feel free to modify to your own personal preference. Whatever you decide to do, have fun with it and love your blend!

Spice Cake Surprise

6 drops cinnamon

6 drops clove oil

5 drops garlic oil

5 drops ginger

Combine all the oils together in a glass jar, or directly into your diffuser. Fill your diffuser with water according to the size of your diffuser.

You can follow the recipe here as is, or you can feel free to modify to your own personal preference. Whatever you decide to do, have fun with it and love your blend!

The Wood Fairies

5 drops rosewood

5 drops cedar wood

8 drops sandalwood

5 drops pine

Combine all the oils together in a glass jar, or directly into your diffuser. Fill your diffuser with water according to the size of your diffuser.

You can follow the recipe here as is, or you can feel free to modify to your own personal preference. Whatever you decide to do, have fun with it and love your blend!

Magic Music

6 drops jasmine

5 drops hyssop

5 drops neem oil

Combine all the oils together in a glass jar, or directly into your diffuser. Fill your diffuser with water according to the size of your diffuser.

You can follow the recipe here as is, or you can feel free to modify to your own personal preference. Whatever you decide to do, have fun with it and love your blend!

The Richness of the Earth

7 drops patchouli

5 drops red cedar

4 drops lemongrass

2 drops rosehip

Combine all the oils together in a glass jar, or directly into your diffuser. Fill your diffuser with water according to the size of your diffuser.

You can follow the recipe here as is, or you can feel free to modify to your own personal preference. Whatever you decide to do, have fun with it and love your blend!

Chapter 3 – Beautiful Day Blends

Few things in life are able to compare to the beauty of a wonderful day. It doesn't need to be anything in particular that makes the day wonderful, but perhaps you are happy to be alive, and you let your happiness overflow into the world around you.

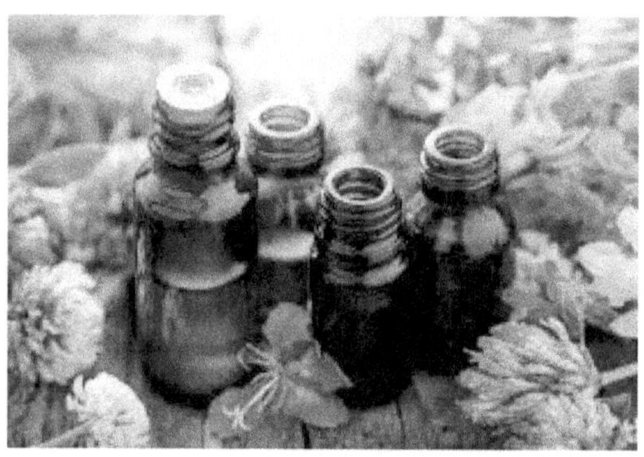

https://www.google.com/search?q=diffuser&espv=2&biw=1366&bih=667&site=webhp&source=lnms&tbm=isch&sa=X&ved=0ahUKEwi2ybOGjvLNAhUHLmMKHbomCEMQ_AUIBygC#imgrc=Rptq34BLaMbFyM%3A

You know that good vibes and happiness are the best things to spread to the world, so why not start with your own home and create a place where good vibes and excellent scents go hand in hand?

You are going to feel as though you escaped to a wonderful fairy garden when you walk into any room of your house, breathing in the deep, crisp scent of any one of these oil blends.

Have fun and let your worries melt away. There is nothing that can compare with these.

Pixels and Pixies

3 drops hibiscus

4 drops rosewood

3 drops basil

3 drops sage

Combine all the oils together in a glass jar, or directly into your diffuser. Fill your diffuser with water according to the size of your diffuser.

You can follow the recipe here as is, or you can feel free to modify to your own personal preference. Whatever you decide to do, have fun with it and love your blend!

A Walk Around The Block

4 drops cedar

4 drops cedarwood

5 drops clary sage

5 drops sage

Combine all the oils together in a glass jar, or directly into your diffuser. Fill your diffuser with water according to the size of your diffuser.

You can follow the recipe here as is, or you can feel free to modify to your own personal preference. Whatever you decide to do, have fun with it and love your blend!

Bees and Butterflies

6 drops spruce

6 drops tangerine

6 drops pine

Combine all the oils together in a glass jar, or directly into your diffuser. Fill your diffuser with water according to the size of your diffuser.

You can follow the recipe here as is, or you can feel free to modify to your own personal preference. Whatever you decide to do, have fun with it and love your blend!

The Gently Blowing Breeze

8 drops patchouli

8 drops lemongrass

4 drops tea tree

5 drops tarragon

Combine all the oils together in a glass jar, or directly into your diffuser. Fill your diffuser with water according to the size of your diffuser.

You can follow the recipe here as is, or you can feel free to modify to your own personal preference. Whatever you decide to do, have fun with it and love your blend!

Fresh Linen on the Line

5 drops peppermint

5 drops eucalyptus

6 drops tangerine

5 drops spearmint

Combine all the oils together in a glass jar, or directly into your diffuser. Fill your diffuser with water according to the size of your diffuser.

You can follow the recipe here as is, or you can feel free to modify to your own personal preference. Whatever you decide to do, have fun with it and love your blend!

Raindrops on the Roses

10 drops eucalyptus

8 drops rosewood

8 drops rose

5 drops sage

Combine all the oils together in a glass jar, or directly into your diffuser. Fill your diffuser with water according to the size of your diffuser.

You can follow the recipe here as is, or you can feel free to modify to your own personal preference. Whatever you decide to do, have fun with it and love your blend!

The Flower Garden

10 drops lavender

10 drops rose

6 drops hibiscus

6 drops lilac

5 drops lemon

5 drops tangerine

Combine all the oils together in a glass jar, or directly into your diffuser. Fill your diffuser with water according to the size of your diffuser.

You can follow the recipe here as is, or you can feel free to modify to your own personal preference. Whatever you decide to do, have fun with it and love your blend!

Umbrella on my Shoulders

10 drops orange

5 drops blood orange

5 drops lime oil

4 drops eucalyptus

Combine all the oils together in a glass jar, or directly into your diffuser. Fill your diffuser with water according to the size of your diffuser.

You can follow the recipe here as is, or you can feel free to modify to your own personal preference. Whatever you decide to do, have fun with it and love your blend!

Chapter 4 – The Best Blends For A Helpful Kick

There's nothing better than a blend that is able to bring life to your house, and fill your house with all kinds of good things in addition to the good vibes you get when you breathe deeply.

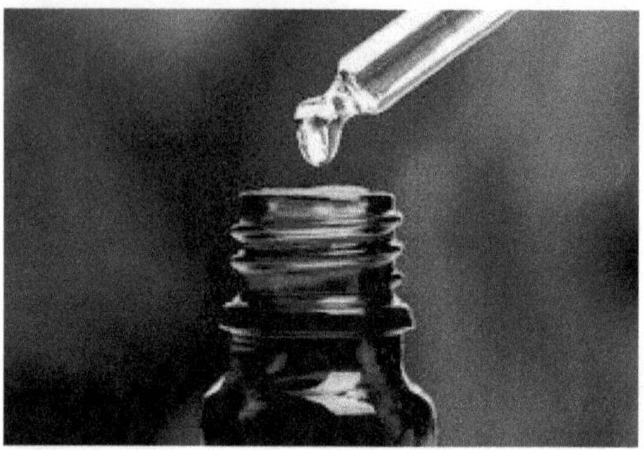

https://www.google.com/search?q=diffuser&espv=2&biw=1366&bih=667&site=webhp&source=lnms&tbm=isch&sa=X&ved=0ahUKEwi2ybOGjvLNAhUH LmMKHbomCEMQ_AUIBygC#imgrc=Rptq34BLaMbFyM%3A

I crafted a blend of the finest scents to bring smiles to your face, but I have also chosen the best oils for headaches, joint pain, and tension. I wanted to fill your home with not only the great, fresh scents that only these oils can bring, but also the peach and relaxation that they possess as well.

When you add these oils to your diffuser, you are combining just what you need to make your home not only delicious and welcoming to all who enter, but you are creating an oasis from the world. A place where you can feel relaxed, pain free, and able to enjoy yourself without any form of tension whatsoever.

So if you want to embrace your own version of a nirvana island, grab your diffuser and these oils, plus a few more of your own if you want to bring in that personal touch.

Toss them into the mix, close your eyes, and sit back to enjoy all of the great benefits of these oils.

The Headache Buster

10 drops peppermint

10 drops eucalyptus

5 drops wintergreen

5 drops spearmint

Combine all the oils together in a glass jar, or directly into your diffuser. Fill your diffuser with water according to the size of your diffuser.

You can follow the recipe here as is, or you can feel free to modify to your own personal preference. Whatever you decide to do, have fun with it and love your blend!

The Immunity Booster

5 drops frankincense

4 drops lemon

4 drops eucalyptus

5 drops garlic

10 drops tea tree

Combine all the oils together in a glass jar, or directly into your diffuser. Fill your diffuser with water according to the size of your diffuser.

You can follow the recipe here as is, or you can feel free to modify to your own personal preference. Whatever you decide to do, have fun with it and love your blend!

The Calming Blend

10 drops vetiver

5 drops lavender

5 drops peppermint

2 drops spearmint

Combine all the oils together in a glass jar, or directly into your diffuser. Fill your diffuser with water according to the size of your diffuser.

You can follow the recipe here as is, or you can feel free to modify to your own personal preference. Whatever you decide to do, have fun with it and love your blend!

The Life of the Party

10 drops lemongrass

4 drops lemon

4 drops tangerine

5 drops sweet orange

5 drops orange

Combine all the oils together in a glass jar, or directly into your diffuser. Fill your diffuser with water according to the size of your diffuser.

You can follow the recipe here as is, or you can feel free to modify to your own personal preference. Whatever you decide to do, have fun with it and love your blend!

The Fixer Fizzer

8 drops tea tree

8 drops peppermint

4 drops myrrh

4 drops cardamom

Combine all the oils together in a glass jar, or directly into your diffuser. Fill your diffuser with water according to the size of your diffuser.

You can follow the recipe here as is, or you can feel free to modify to your own personal preference. Whatever you decide to do, have fun with it and love your blend!

The All In One Blend

5 drops goldenseal

10 drops grapefruit

4 drops ginger

4 drops cinnamon

Combine all the oils together in a glass jar, or directly into your diffuser. Fill your diffuser with water according to the size of your diffuser.

You can follow the recipe here as is, or you can feel free to modify to your own personal preference. Whatever you decide to do, have fun with it and love your blend!

Aches and Pains Melt Away Blend

11 drops lavender

11 drops spruce

5 drops cedar wood

5 drops grapefruit

Combine all the oils together in a glass jar, or directly into your diffuser. Fill your diffuser with water according to the size of your diffuser.

You can follow the recipe here as is, or you can feel free to modify to your own personal preference. Whatever you decide to do, have fun with it and love your blend!

The Bedroom Blend

10 drops peppermint

5 drops cinnamon

5 drops wintergreen

5 drops spruce

Combine all the oils together in a glass jar, or directly into your diffuser. Fill your diffuser with water according to the size of your diffuser.

You can follow the recipe here as is, or you can feel free to modify to your own personal preference. Whatever you decide to do, have fun with it and love your blend!

Chapter 5 – Unique Blends For The Uniquely You

The best way to describe any of the blends in this chapter is with the word unique. There is something simply delightful but entirely one of a kind about each of the blends, and I highly encourage you to add your little touch of personality to any or all of them.

Have fun with it, use your imagination, and use as little or as much of any of the oils as you wish. If you think that there's another little something that would bring out the right note, toss it into the mix!

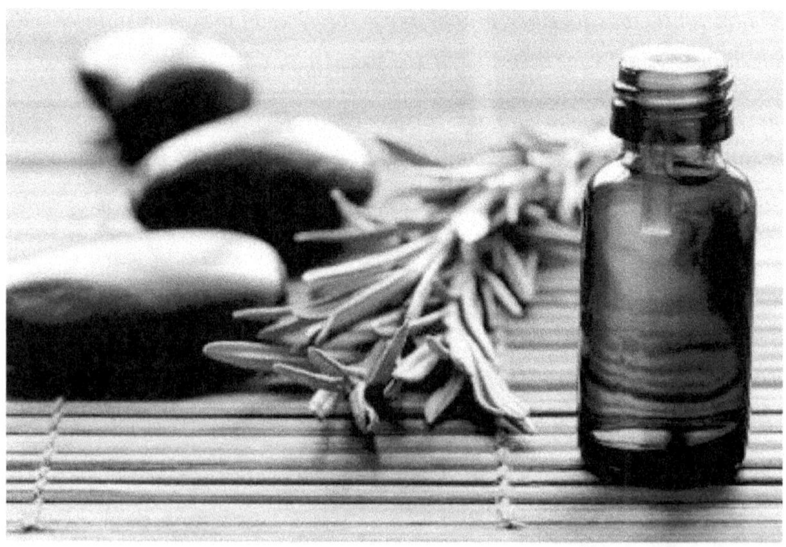

https://www.google.com/search?
q=diffuser&espv=2&biw=1366&bih=667&site=webhp&source=lnms&tbm=isch&sa=X&ved=0ahUKEwi2ybOGjvLNAhUH
LmMKHbomCEMQ_AUIBygC#imgrc=Rptq34BLaMbFyM%3A

You can't go wrong with it, and if you are in love, then the blend is the perfect blend for you.

Just What You Needed Blend

8 drops cinnamon

7 drops orange

5 drops patchouli

3 drops spruce

Combine all the oils together in a glass jar, or directly into your diffuser. Fill your diffuser with water according to the size of your diffuser.

You can follow the recipe here as is, or you can feel free to modify to your own personal preference. Whatever you decide to do, have fun with it and love your blend!

Yours Truly Blend

10 drops rose

8 drops lavender

3 drops spearmint

3 drops grapefruit

3 drops tea tree oil

Combine all the oils together in a glass jar, or directly into your diffuser. Fill your diffuser with water according to the size of your diffuser.

You can follow the recipe here as is, or you can feel free to modify to your own personal preference. Whatever you decide to do, have fun with it and love your blend!

Anything and Everything

8 drops frankincense

4 drops spikenard

4 drops patchouli

4 drops vetiver

3 drops spruce

Combine all the oils together in a glass jar, or directly into your diffuser. Fill your diffuser with water according to the size of your diffuser.

You can follow the recipe here as is, or you can feel free to modify to your own personal preference. Whatever you decide to do, have fun with it and love your blend!

Everything You Wanted Blend

9 drops ylang ylang

5 drops tangerine

5 drops wintergreen

4 drops cedar wood

Combine all the oils together in a glass jar, or directly into your diffuser. Fill your diffuser with water according to the size of your diffuser.

You can follow the recipe here as is, or you can feel free to modify to your own personal preference. Whatever you decide to do, have fun with it and love your blend!

You and Me is Three Blend

4 drops tea tree

8 drops grapefruit

8 drops cinnamon

Combine all the oils together in a glass jar, or directly into your diffuser. Fill your diffuser with water according to the size of your diffuser.

You can follow the recipe here as is, or you can feel free to modify to your own personal preference. Whatever you decide to do, have fun with it and love your blend!

Your Dream Come True Blend

8 drops lavender

9 drops spruce

4 drops ylang ylang

3 drops tea tree

Combine all the oils together in a glass jar, or directly into your diffuser. Fill your diffuser with water according to the size of your diffuser.

You can follow the recipe here as is, or you can feel free to modify to your own personal preference. Whatever you decide to do, have fun with it and love your blend!

The Super Spoiler Blend

12 drops ylang ylang

6 drops vetiver

4 drops myrrh

4 drops patchouli

Combine all the oils together in a glass jar, or directly into your diffuser. Fill your diffuser with water according to the size of your diffuser.

You can follow the recipe here as is, or you can feel free to modify to your own personal preference. Whatever you decide to do, have fun with it and love your blend!

Indulgence in Love Blend

7 drops cinnamon

4 drops rose

4 drops tangerine

2 drops spearmint

2 drops tea tree oil

Combine all the oils together in a glass jar, or directly into your diffuser. Fill your diffuser with water according to the size of your diffuser.

You can follow the recipe here as is, or you can feel free to modify to your own personal preference. Whatever you decide to do, have fun with it and love your blend!

Conclusion

There you have it, everything you need to know to make the best blends for your diffuser any time you want. Whether you are creating a blend that is going to be for relaxation, to help with your mood, or to set the tone for the day, you will have everything you need in this book.

I hope this book was able to show you how many different blends you can use, how to make the best blends for your needs, and how to use blends to make the results you want to see.

It doesn't matter how many oils you have, the size of your diffuser, or the amount you want to use, there's no way you can overdo. Have fun and use the different blends I have put together for you, or have fun and create your own.

The more you explore, the more fun you are going to have creating your own blends. These recipes are the perfect solution to any kind of day you are having. Use them to relax and enhance your day, use them to make your day even better, or use them to bring a bad day to the right side of things.

No matter how you want to do it, you are going to have just what you need with these essential oil blends, and in no time at all your home is going to be full of the deliciousness that you have been yearning for.

So what are you waiting for? There is a whole new world out there for you to dive into and enjoy, and that is just what this book is going to help you jump in to. No matter how much experience you have, how many oils you have, or how many times you have tried this before, these oils are going to be the best of the best for your day.

Grab a few bottles, crack open your diffuser, and you are going to fall in love with the different options you have. All that you have to do now is sit back and relax, and enjoy all the wonderful things you will experience from these incredible blends.

Get ready to indulge in every kind of pampering you like, and you will reap all of the wonderful benefits that come from the use of essential oils.

Your oasis awaits, jump on in and enjoy.

FREE Bonus Reminder

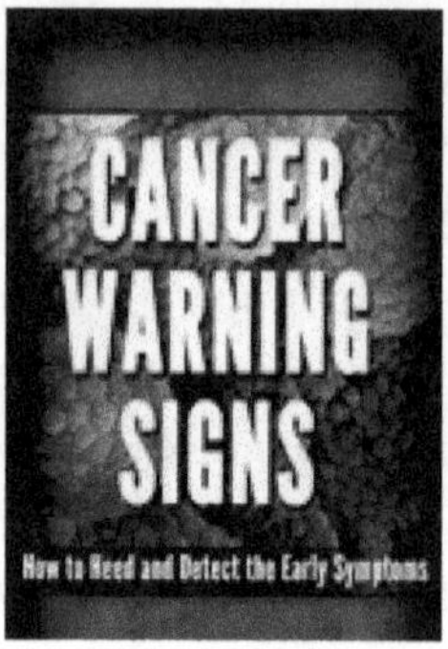

If you have not grabbed it yet, please go ahead and download your special bonus report *"DIY Projects. 13 Useful & Easy To Make DIY Projects To Save Money & Improve Your Home!"*

Simply Click the Button Below

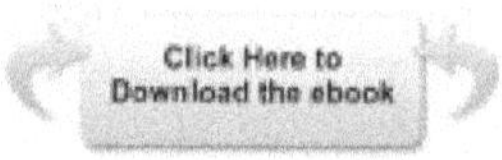

OR Go to This Page

http://healthylivingpeople.com/free/

BONUS #2: More Free & Discounted Books

Do you want to receive more Free & Discounted Books?

We have a mailing list where we send out our new Books when they go free or with a discount on Kindle. Click on the link below to sign up for Free & Discount Book Promotions.

=> Sign Up for Free & Discount Book Promotions <=

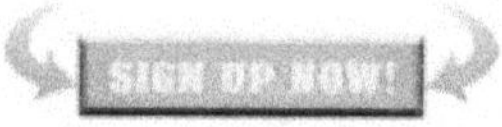

OR Go to this URL

http://zbit.ly/1WBb1Ek

www.ingramcontent.com/pod-product-compliance
Lightning Source LLC
Chambersburg PA
CBHW050803240726
48654CB00008B/610